Kick Out Childhood Obesity

How to Overcome Childhood Obesity with Food and Simple Home Remedies

By

Bradley T. Macfarlane

Copyright © by **Bradley T. Macfarlane 2023**

All rights reserved. Before this document is

Duplicated or reproduced in any manner, the publisher's consent must be obtained.

Therefore, the contents within cannot be stored electronically, transferred, or kept in a database.

Neither in part nor in full can the document be copied, scanned, faxed, or retained without approval from the publisher or creator.

TABLE OF CONTENTS

Introduction

Obesity in childhood is a major medical problem that affects children and adolescents. It's especially concerning because excess pounds frequently set children on the path to health problems that were long considered adult issues, such as diabetes, high blood pressure, and high cholesterol.

Obesity in childhood can also lead to low self-esteem and depression. Improving your entire family's food and exercise habits is one of the most effective techniques for reducing childhood obesity.

Childhood obesity treatment and prevention protect your child's health now and in the future. Childhood obesity has emerged as one of the most serious medical and public health issues of our day.

Childhood obesity is linked to a number of comorbidities that have an impact on both physical and mental health.

Chapter 1

What causes childhood obesity?

Obesity in children is a complicated condition with many underlying causes. It's not due to indolence or a lack of courage, either. Your youngster needs a specific number of calories for growth and development.

People's bodies store extra calories as fat when they consume more calories than they expend. The same factors that cause adults to gain weight also affect children. There are many causes of childhood obesity, including:

Behavior

Shared family behaviors, such as eating habits and being inactive, can contribute to childhood obesity. The balance of calories consumed with calories burned plays a role in determining your child's weight.

Busy families are consuming more foods and beverages high in fat, sugar, and calories. These foods and beverages tend to be low in vitamins, minerals, and other vital nutrients.

At the same time, many children are spending less time outdoors and more time indoors being inactive. As video games, tablets, and smartphones continue to grow in popularity, the number of hours of inactivity may only increase.

If you inherit genes that place you at a higher risk for obesity, developing a family environment that models appropriate diet and exercise practices will help you overcome the genetic tendency for obesity. Family dynamics and home environment are regarded as having an even greater impact on weight than genetics.

The more convenient, low-calorie, and nutrient-dense foods there are at home, the more likely your family will eat them. And if you want your children to eat more fruits and vegetables, be sure that mom and dad eat them as well. Consider performing a healthy kitchen makeover. Start by evaluating if fruits and vegetables are easily accessible in your home. Do you keep fruits and vegetables washed, cut, and ready to eat in your fridge?

The community and social and economic status

Shared family behaviors, such as eating habits and being inactive, can contribute to childhood obesity. The balance of calories consumed with calories burned plays a role in determining your child's weight.

Busy families are consuming more foods and beverages high in fat, sugar, and calories. These foods and beverages tend to be low in vitamins, minerals, and other vital nutrients.

At the same time, many children are spending less time outdoors and more time indoors being inactive. As video games, tablets, and smartphones continue to grow in popularity, the number of hours of inactivity may only increase. Obesity in children has reached dangerous levels. Despite the fact that this pandemic affects people of various socioeconomic, racial, and ethnic backgrounds, the trend is more common among kids from lower socioeconomic homes.

The reasons for this disparity in obesity rates by socioeconomic status include a variety of factors, such as the accessibility of safer places for physical activity as well as disparities in the availability of healthier meals in families and schools.

Increases in type 2 diabetes diagnoses across some ethnic groups and differences in the accessibility of health care for kids from poorer socioeconomic backgrounds are both alarming trends.

It will be crucial to focus on children from lower socioeconomic backgrounds as our society works to enhance our children's lifestyles and reduce obesity rates.

Genetic factors

There may be a genetic predisposition to childhood obesity. Children are more likely to get the condition themselves if their parents or other family members are fat. Studies have connected a number of genes to weight gain.

 Childhood obesity is predicted by parental obesity. When a parent is fat, the familial risk ratio for childhood obesity exceeds 2.5. With considerable maternal and paternal impacts in addition to the neonatal genes, birth weight is characterized by a genetic heritability component of around 30%.

About five of these genes have been identified, and they account for about 5% of cases of childhood obesity. PraderWilli syndrome (PWS), a hereditary disease brought on by chromosomal abnormalities, is an illustration of the genetic etiology of obesity. People who have PWS experience central nervous system malfunction, which causes unusually high appetites and early-onset obesity.

Cultural Factors

Childhood obesity can be increased by advertisements for fast food restaurants and harmful snack foods. Children watch advertisements on television and on billboards in their areas.

These items are frequently high in calories and/or available in huge quantities. These variables may all contribute to childhood obesity.

Hormonal abnormalities are another risk factor for childhood obesity. On the other hand, illnesses are rarely the root of childhood obesity. Any medical issues will be ruled out through a physical examination and maybe blood tests.

Some medications can increase the likelihood of gaining weight or being obese. Several ethnic parents were less worried about the potential repercussions of childhood obesity and saw a greater body size as desirable. This may be because in some cultures, being overweight is associated with prosperity and good health, which can make some parents desire to "feed up" their kids.

Parents from particular ethnic backgrounds place a greater importance on academic and cultural education than physical education, which can leave little time for physical activity after attending church schools, taking language classes, and doing homework.

Chapter 2

Diets for treating childhood obesity

Your child may put on weight if they consume high-calorie items on a regular basis, like fast food, baked goods, and vending machine snacks.

Candy and desserts can also contribute to weight gain, and mounting evidence implicates sugary beverages, such as fruit juices and sports drinks, in the development of obesity in some individuals.

We keep our meals delicious and exciting by eating a variety of foods. Each food includes a special blend of nutrients, including macronutrients (carbohydrate, protein, and fat) and micronutrients (vitamins and minerals), making it essential to a healthy and balanced diet.

A guideline for making optimal dietary decisions is provided by The Kid's Healthy Eating Plate.

Divide the remaining half of the plate equally between whole grains and lean protein, and fill half of it with colorful vegetables and fruits (and choose them as snacks).
A healthy diet should include plenty of fruits and vegetables, but diversity is just as important as quantity. You cannot obtain all the nutrients you need for good health from just one fruit or vegetable. Each day, eat a lot.

This not only ensures a wider range of Consuming plenty of fruits and vegetables helps lower blood pressure, reduce the risk of heart disease and stroke, protect against some types of cancer, improve blood sugar levels, which can help regulate appetite, and reduce the risk of eye and digestive problems.

Non-starchy fruits and vegetables, including apples, pears, and green leafy vegetables, should be consumed in order to avoid weight gain. Its low glycemic index This not only ensures a wider range of Consuming plenty of fruits and vegetables helps lower blood pressure, reduce the risk of heart disease and stroke, protect against some types of cancer, improve blood sugar levels, which can help regulate appetite, and reduce the risk of eye and digestive problems.

Choose whole-grain cereals instead of processed ones.

 In contrast to refined grains, which are depleted of important nutrients during the refining process, whole grains provide a "complete package" of health advantages. The endosperm, the germ, and the bra are the three components that make up each whole grain kernel

. Health-improving nutrients are contained in each segment. The outer, fiber-rich layer known as the bran contains antioxidants, phytochemicals, B vitamins, iron, copper, zinc, and magnesium. Plants naturally contain substances called phytochemicals, which have been studied for their potential to prevent disease. The embryo, the middle of the seed where fertilization takes place, is a rich source of phytochemicals, antioxidants, vitamin E, and healthy fats. The inner layer, or endosperm, contains protein, carbs, and trace amounts of several vitamins and minerals.

The effects of these elements on our bodies are varied. Bran and fiber prevent rapid rises in insulin levels by reducing how quickly starch breaks down into glucose. Fiber facilitates the collective of waste material through the gastrointestinal system and lowers cholesterol.

 Additionally, fiber may assist in preventing the development of tiny blood clots that can result in heart attacks or strokes. Whole grains contain phytochemicals and important minerals, including magnesium, selenium, and copper, that may help prevent some malignancies.

The way we process grains has altered since the invention of industrialized rolling mills in the latter part of the nineteenth century. Both the germ and the bran are removed during milling, leaving only the endosperm, which is soft and simple to digest. The grain is simpler to break down after the tough bran is removed. The removal of the germ is done to extend the shelf life of processed wheat products since the germ contains fat. Cereals that are extremely refined have substantially poorer nutritional quality.

Wheat is refined to produce puffy flour that produces light, airy breads and pastries, but during the process, more than half of the B vitamins, 90% of the vitamin E, and nearly all of the fiber are removed.

 Despite the fact that fortification can restore some nutrients, it cannot replace whole grains' other health-promoting ingredients, like phytochemicals.
A growing body of evidence demonstrates that reducing consumption of refined grains and adopting whole grain products as well as other less-processed, higher-quality sources of carbs enhances health in a variety of ways.

Healthy Protein Foods

When possible, get your protein from plants. Eating nuts, seeds, whole grains, legumes (beans and peas), and other plant-based sources of protein is good for both your health and the health of the environment.

Make sure to vary your protein sources if the majority of your intake comes from plants to ensure that no "essential" protein components are missed.

The good news is that there are many alternatives to mix and match within the plant kingdom. Here are a few illustrations from each category:

Lentils, beans (adzuki, black, fava, chickpeas/garbanzo, kidney, etc.), peas (green, snow, snap, split, etc.), soybeans (and soy-derived products: tofu, tempeh, etc.), and peanuts are examples of legumes.

Almonds, pistachios, cashews, walnuts, hazelnuts, pecans, hemp seeds, pumpkin and squash seeds, sunflower seeds, flax seeds, sesame seeds, and chia seeds are some examples of nuts and seeds.

Wheat, quinoa, wild rice, millet, oats, and buckwheat are examples of whole grains.

Other: While many fruits and vegetables include some protein, it is often present in lower concentrations than in other plant-based diets.

Corn, broccoli, and other produce are a few examples of foods with higher protein content levels.

Improve your animal protein sources. When it comes to diets containing animal products, taking into account the protein package is particularly crucial.

Your best bets are typically seafood (fish, crustaceans, and mollusks) and fowl (chicken, turkey, and duck). Another nice option is eggs.

It's advisable to consume dairy products in moderation if you like them (aim for 1-2 servings per day; yogurt is probably a better option than obtaining all of your servings from milk or cheese).

Red meat should only be eaten in moderation, which includes unprocessed beef, hog, lamb, veal, mutton, and goat meat. If you prefer red meat, think about eating it in moderation or just on exceptional occasions.

Avoid processed meats like bacon, hot dogs, sausages, and cold cuts. Processed meats also include foods like turkey bacon, chicken sausage, and deli-sliced chicken and ham, despite the fact that these products are frequently derived from red meats.

Meat that has been "transformed through salting, curing, fermentation, smoking, or other processes to enhance flavor or improve preservation" is referred to as processed meat.

Uncertain of where to begin in your efforts to cut back on red and processed meats

Here are a few tips for making savings while still cooking great, filling meals. Just locate your "starting point" and proceed.

Healthy oil and Fats

Additionally, it's critical to keep in mind that while fat is a vital component of our diet, the kind of fat we consume is what really counts. We should restrict foods high in saturated fat

 (especially red meat), consistently choose foods with healthy unsaturated fats (such as fish, nuts, seeds, and healthy oils from plants), and steer clear of unhealthy Tran's fats (from partly hydrogenated oils).
Use extra virgin olive oil, canola oil, corn oil, sunflower oil, and peanut oil as healthy plant oils in cooking, on salads and vegetables, and at the table. Use butter only sometimes.

The kind of fat you consume is most important when it comes to dietary fat. Compared to earlier dietary advice that advocated low-fat diets, more recent research demonstrates that good fats are essential and advantageous for health.

Vegetable oils (including olive, canola, sunflower, soy, and corn oils), nuts, seeds, and fish are among the foods high in healthy fats.

Chapter 3

Inadequate physical activity

Because they don't burn as many calories, kids who don't exercise a lot are more likely to gain weight. The issue is further exacerbated by spending too much time doing sedentary activities like watching television or playing video games.

TV programs frequently include commercials for harmful meals. Children and teenagers should strive to engage in at least one hour of physical activity each day, without the use of expensive equipment or a gym.

Kick Out Childhood Obesity

According to the Physical Activity Guidelines for Americans, kids should engage in unstructured activities like tug-of-war or playground games.

Although a lot of people think of exercise as a technique to reduce weight, it is important for the body's overall health. Worldwide, a significant portion of children struggle with obesity. One of the main reasons for childhood obesity is parents' lack of concern for their children's nutrition and, specifically, their lack of physical activity.

Doctors claim that obesity is a global problem, particularly at this time when children's physical activities have been substituted by using technology.

Worldwide, a significant portion of children struggle with obesity. One of the main reasons for childhood obesity is parents' lack of concern for their children's nutrition and, specifically, their lack of physical activity.

Doctors claim that obesity is a global problem, particularly at this time when children's physical activities have been substituted by using technology.

When a person is less active, they frequently acquire weight, regardless of age. Exercise helps you maintain a healthy weight by burning calories.

Sports, time on the playground, and other physical activities can help kids burn more calories, but if they aren't encouraged to do so, they may not do as well.

Children can benefit from physical activity in a number of ways, such as:

- maintaining a healthy weight
- Increased cardiovascular fitness (heart and lungs).
- Better posture.
- Improved sleeping habits.
- A rise in confidence and self-esteem
- Increased ability to focus.
- Support relaxation.
- Strengthening bones and muscles.

Early physical exercise introduction for your Child

Support your child's desire for exercise whenever you can. For instance, kick the ball with them when they ask.

Teach your child the fundamentals of sportsmanship, such as how to leap, skip, and throw a ball. According to research, kids with weak fundamental skills tend to steer clear of sports.

Bring them to the neighborhood playground and assist them in using the apparatus. Have a try yourself; slides and swings are entertaining, and if you are having a good time, your youngster will likely play with you for longer.

Try out various sports in classes with other people your age. Gymnastics, football, and dancing are just a few of the activities that have been modified for young children.

Make sure part of your family's outings involves exercise.

Engage your child in physical household chores like gardening, car washing, or housecleaning. Instead of driving short distances, consider walking. Students should be encouraged to use bicycles or walk to school.

Take your toddler for routine neighborhood strolls. Young children and infants can be transported in strollers; as they get bigger, encourage them to walk some of the distance. Alternatives to organized exercise for families with children

Physical activity has numerous advantages for health and wellbeing that go beyond scheduled events.

The following are some enjoyable family activities that don't feel like exercise:

1. Kite-flying in a park or on a beach

2. Dancing to your preferred tunes

3. Cycling alongside the river or on designated bike paths

4. Playing a game of table tennis with the family

5. Splashing around and swimming at the neighborhood pool

6. Walking the dog.

7. Frisbee throwing

8. Skateboarding, rollerblading, or other similar activities require everyone to wear the proper safety gear.

9. Trampoline jumping

Children's physical activities during the winter

On bright days, it's easy to be active, but throughout the winter, most of us choose to stay inside. The following are some ideas for remaining active during the winter:

On chilly, rainy days, wrap up and go outside. Give your youngster the chance to experience how different seasons affect locations like the beach. It's enjoyable to splash through puddles. Put on raincoats and gumboots, and then jump through puddles with your kid.

Indoor sports, including swimming, trampoline jumping, table tennis, and cricket, are just a few examples. Investigate several choices in your neighborhood. Some sports, such as Australian Rules football, are traditionally played during the winter months.

Chapter 4

Psychological aspects

Stress on the individual, the parents, and the family might raise a child's risk of obesity. Some kids binge eat to deal with issues, manage emotions like stress, or get rid of boredom.

Similar characteristics in their parents may exist. When, when, and how food and beverages are consumed are referred to as eating behaviors or habits.

Children with inappropriate eating habits consume too much energy, and their diets lack the nutrients they need for healthy development.

Such unhealthy eating practices include, for instance, grazing on highly processed and calorie-dense foods between meals. Dining in front of the TV, skipping breakfast, and consuming sugary beverages

Beverages with added sugar, frequent dining out, and emotional eating.

Poor eating habits are a major contributor to the emergence of obesity. Early childhood is often when eating habits are developed, and parents have a significant impact on this process.

In order to lower the risk of adult overweight, obesity, and cardiovascular disease, parents and other caregivers can play a vital role in fostering an environment that encourages children to develop healthier eating habits early in life.

Instead of focusing on restricting children's choices or emphasizing body weight, parents and caregivers should create an environment that supports and promotes healthy dietary choices. Parents and other adults who are responsible for children should:

Meals should be served at regular intervals, and children should be allowed to choose from a variety of nutritious options. Nutritious or novel foods should be served alongside favorites.

- Routinely trying out new, healthy foods with the child and showing them how much you like them;

- Observing a child's verbal or nonverbal signals of hunger and fullness; and

- Not forcing kids to eat more than they want to eat

Allowing kids to make their own food choices can be difficult for some parents and caregivers, especially if the kids start to become picky eaters or are unwilling to try new foods.

Between the ages of one and five, when toddlers are first discovering the flavors and textures of solid foods, these behaviors are frequent and accepted as typical. It may seem like a good idea in the short run to impose strict, authoritarian restrictions over what may and cannot be eaten, along with applying incentives or sanctions.

Research, however, does not support this strategy; on the contrary, it might have unfavorable long-term effects. An authoritarian eating environment prevents a child from developing good decision-making abilities and may diminish their sense of control, both of which are critical stages in a child's development.

Additionally, the authoritarian approach has been connected to children eating when they are not hungry and consuming less healthful, likely calorie-dense foods. This could increase the risk of becoming overweight, obese, and/or having eating disorders.

However, allowing a child to eat everything they want whenever they want without any restriction does not set up enough boundaries for kids to form good eating habits. Additionally, research has connected this strategy to a higher risk of youngsters becoming overweight or obese.

If a youngster is "picky" or "fussy" about food, research does indicate that several measures can boost their dietary variety during their early years. Children are more likely to accept healthy foods if they are frequently offered a range of them, especially if they are accompanied by items they already enjoy.

Furthermore, caregivers or parents who eat a food joyfully may help a youngster accept it. To encourage kids to be open to a wider variety of food alternatives, caregivers, siblings, and peers can set a good example by consuming healthful foods.

Since many different people in a child's life have an impact on their eating habits, a healthy diet should be practiced by the entire family. It's crucial to remember that not every strategy will work for every child, and parents and other caregivers shouldn't feel overly stressed or responsible for their kids' eating habits.

Kick Out Childhood Obesity

"It is obvious that every child is unique and has a different propensity to grow into a person who makes healthy dietary choices. This is why it's crucial to put more effort into developing an atmosphere that promotes decision-making abilities and exposes kids to a variety of healthy, nutritious foods throughout childhood, rather than giving the child's choices too much attention.

Eat as many meals as you can as a family and serve a range of healthy dishes. Encourage children to consume five servings of fruits and vegetables each day, as well as breakfast each day, and to avoid drinking too much sugar-sweetened liquid, such as soda, juice, and sports drinks. Make certain they get adequate rest.

Building trust and removing any stigma associated with obesity can be accomplished by discussing it openly rather than avoiding it. Children want their parents to tell them whether they are overweight or not and to support their efforts to lead healthy lives. . For instance, discuss how good eating, rest, and exercise can improve one's overall health and inevitably aid in weight loss. Leading a healthier lifestyle can aid them in making more informed decisions.

Chapter 5

Risk signs of childhood obesity

Childhood obesity is the most challenging issue in public health in the twenty-first century. It is currently acknowledged as a worldwide pandemic health problem. Fatty children are more likely to be diagnosed with diabetes and heart problems early in life and are more likely to stay fat as adults.

Children who are obese have greater rates of mortality and morbidity. In light of the current situation, reducing childhood obesity is of utmost importance. Body mass index (BMI), which calculates a person's weight in relation to their height, is a recognized indication of overweight and obesity.

By using growth charts, the BMI, and, if necessary, additional tests, your child's doctor can assist you in determining whether your child's weight could result in health issues.

Speak with your child's doctor if you are concerned that they are gaining too much weight. Your child's growth and development history, your family's history of weight for height, and where your child ranks on the growth charts will all be taken into account by the doctor.

This might aid in figuring out whether your child's weight is within unhealthy bounds. A child's physical, social, and emotional wellbeing can be impacted by childhood obesity on a regular basis.

The physical complications of childhood obesity may

Include:

- **Diabetes type 2** The way your child's body uses sugar (glucose) is impacted by this chronic disease. The risk of type 2 diabetes is increased by obesity and a sedentary lifestyle.

- **High blood pressure and cholesterol**. Your child may develop one or both of these illnesses as a result of a bad diet. These elements may help plaque accumulate in the arteries, which may restrict and harden the arteries later in life, possibly resulting in a heart attack or stroke.

- **Joint ache**. Additional weight puts additional strain on the knees and hips. Hips, knees, and back pain are two common side effects of childhood obesity.

- **Breathing difficulties**. Children who are overweight are more likely to have asthma. Additionally, these kids are more likely to be affected by obstructive sleep apnea, a potentially dangerous condition when a child's breathing continuously pauses and resumes as they sleep.

Issues of a societal and behavioral nature

Children who are obese may be teased or bullied by their classmates. Loss of self-esteem and an elevated risk of sadness and anxiety can follow from this. It takes more than just feeling down or having a terrible day to be depressed.

 You may be depressed if a depressive state persists for a long time and interferes with daily activities.

Symptoms of depression include

Having difficulties sleeping or staying asleep; not wanting to engage in activities that used to be enjoyable; feeling irritated, easily annoyed, or restless

- Getting up too early or staying up late Eating more or less than usual or not feeling hungry

- Aches, pains, headaches, or gastrointestinal issues that don't get better with treatment: decide what to do.

- Feeling exhausted despite getting enough rest

- Guilt, worthlessness, or helplessness

- Considering harming yourself or taking your own life

If your child has anxiety, certain triggers may cause them to experience acute and uncontrollable terror. They could worry about the future or experience terrifying panic attacks marked by a racing heart and difficulty breathing. The majority of the time, a depressed child may experience sadness and irritability.

If anxiety problems aren't adequately treated, they can become chronic, just like other illnesses. The majority of children discover that they require expert coaching to effectively manage and overcome their anxiety. Children with anxiety problems can get a variety of treatments that have been scientifically demonstrated to be efficient.

Conclusion

Obesity in children is a possibility when they consume too many calories and don't exercise or sleep enough. Some kids might only have sporadic access to wholesome foods like fruits and vegetables.

This covers residents of low-income areas. Many kids don't engage in enough exercise. There are more kids watching TV, playing video games, and engaging in other screen-related activities, which is why parents can transform kids' lives for the better by doing the following:

Make your family move more. All day long, children ages 3 to 5 should be engaged in physical activity.

This includes sports like skipping and riding a tricycle. Children between the ages of 6 and 17 should engage in 60 minutes or more of medium- to high-intensity physical activity each day.

This can incorporate entertaining aerobic exercises like tag and rope jumping. By staying active yourself, you may set a good example for your kids. Include physical activity in your everyday routine.

As often as you can, try going on family walks, dancing, riding, or playing a game outside.

Create a consistent sleep schedule. Sound sleep aids in disease prevention. Type 2 diabetes, obesity, accidents, and issues with attention and conduct are a few of these. Lack of sleep in children increases their chance of gaining weight unhealthily.

Take all the screens out of your kid's room. Screen use should be stopped at least an hour before bed. Maintain a regular sleeping schedule, even on the weekends. This may improve sleep for kids.

Set an example of a balanced diet. Children can achieve and maintain a healthy weight by eating a better diet as a family. **In order to prevent childhood obesity, parents should assist their children.**

THE END

www.ingramcontent.com/pod-product-compliance
Lightning Source LLC
Chambersburg PA
CBHW080947260726
48661CB00010B/4127